When the Red Arrow Points Up: A Guide Toward the Cost of Wellness at Work

Michelle Greene Rhodes

MHS, RN, CCM, CMCN

Table of Contents

Introduction

*"An empty lantern provides no light. Self-care is the fuel that allows your light to shine brightly." ~ **Unknown***

Welcome to the definitive guide on transforming your organization through self-care. Before we get started, let's make one thing resoundingly clear. In my profession, I meet lots of people, and their initial feelings on self-care all echo the same message. That message is: *Self-care is selfish, and if I make it a priority, then I am selfish.*

I want to properly dispel this myth. Self-care has nothing to do with selfishness, though both do contain the word, "self." Over the years, I believe self-care has been conflated with the concept of treating yourself, but self-care is not about buying fancy green juices and spending hours of your life getting the latest luxury treatment. It's not about wiling away your time in expensive stores looking for a new bag for the season or scheduling weekly appointments at a half dozen different salons.

Self-care is a mindset. It's an approach to life where you respect yourself enough to make sure that you're getting what you need when you need it, just like you ensure that your family is getting the things that they need when it matters. Somehow though in our society, it's fine and even encouraged, to put the needs of loved ones ahead of her own. It's looked at favorably if you sacrifice a new pair of walking sneakers for yourself so that your husband has a new tie to wear to work or to even sacrifice the hour when you would walk around the neighborhood to bring your kids to the mall. Of course, there are always instances when you'll have to weigh two options against each other and make the reasonable decision.

But the current that should run beneath all of your decisions is a dedication to self-care. Self-care will give you the stamina to care for others and live your best life. So the meaning of self-care that I'm going to challenge you to take on and live is this one. Self-care means having a healthy relationship with yourself so that you can nurture others from a place of strength and confidence. True self-care isn't about whether you just had the most expensive manicure or not. It's about establishing healthy boundaries between yourself and those closest to you. It's about honesty, with yourself and with those around you, it's about eliminating toxins from your system that do your body harm and only serve to drown out the pain you feel inside. And it's about addressing old traumas and moving forward toward healing, self-respect and love.

You'll be surprised too. The amazing thing that happens when you start focusing on self-care is that you will need others to take of you less. You won't be reliant on others to get your needs met because you will be meeting these needs yourself. You will no longer be vulnerable or waiting to be appreciated for all that you do. At first, this might sound like the opposite of what you want. You might be thinking, "I always help others, shouldn't someone want to help me for a change and isn't that how I know that I am loved or cared for?"

It might seem counterintuitive, but that answer is, "no." When you practice self-care, you will become confident because you will see that your well-being is totally under your control. That puts you in the driver's seat. You're not waiting for scraps of appreciation from anyone else. You are strong on your own. You don't need love the same way you did before you had it for yourself. Instead you want it, but it's extra, it's not required to make you feel worthy. If you're starving for food, then you need the next meal, regardless of what it is because you're that hungry. When you're so hungry for anything, you lose the ability of choice and desire. But if you're satisfied with what you have already, and someone offers you a sundae, it's a treat or a gift. You have what you need, and now you have even more.

Once you are immersed in healthy practices of self-care, those same people you were hoping would appreciate you will either start to respect you more and crave to be around you, or they will fall away because they no longer have any power or control over you. Whatever the result, you are enough all on your own. You are in control of the only things which you can control, your own behaviors, actions and mindsets. And the things out of your control, namely other people's decisions, actions and mindsets don't affect you in the debilitating way they can affect if you if your are relying on others for your sense of self and well being.

Everything you need to live a healthy and satisfying life is within you already. And once you start practicing true self-care, you'll have even more energy and love to share with others. When you feel good about yourself and are in a good and healthy place, that light can't help but to spill out onto everyone in your orbit. This includes coworkers and the workplace culture.

When your self-esteem is low, you can't help but gravitate toward people also on that lower plane. And if you don't feel confident in yourself and your abilities, you will constantly look outside yourself to be affirmed. Sometimes you might get it, but because the giving is not coming from within, it won't be consistent. You'll always be at the mercy of what others think about you or how they act toward you.

Instead, it is time to nurture your inner joy so as to attract more it. It's time to focus on strengthening your mind, body and spirit so that you can live the live that you were meant to live. You are doing the world a disservice if you are not living your best life. You are not here on this earth to sacrifice your own needs or to tread so lightly that you don't cause others pain. You're meant to be who you are in every way possible. Only then can you truly help others. If you want to be a positive influence in the world, you simply must have a self-care practice. Having value for yourself first will allow you to truly value others in ways that are healthy for them as well.

This book is divided into three sections, the Mind, the Body and the Spirit. Within those sections are chapters on smaller areas within those bigger categories. I'll share with you some ways to focus on self-care in these areas, and then we're going to put a price tag on these things. That price is what you will pay if you neglect these elements of your life. It's up to you whether this cost is worth it or not. I'm willing to bet if you've made it this far, that you're already thinking it's definitely not and that you're ready for change. I'll also leave you with a few questions to ask yourself that can help propel you into action on a this newfound journey of self-care.

I will help you cultivate a practice of self-care in your life that will leave you feeling like 100 times the woman you already are. I'm sure that you're already giving so much to those around you, but I bet you're giving from a place of feeling tired and spent. When you incorporate self-care into your world, you will expand beyond anything you can imagine. You will feel like nothing can stop you, because it can't. When you have self-love, you are unvanquishable. You can never again be made to feel small, because your feeling small is not up to anyone but you. By the end of this book, you'll even understand why striving to see yourself as powerful, whole and loved is the only approach that makes sense.

Now, let's get ready to start on this journey. Are you with me?

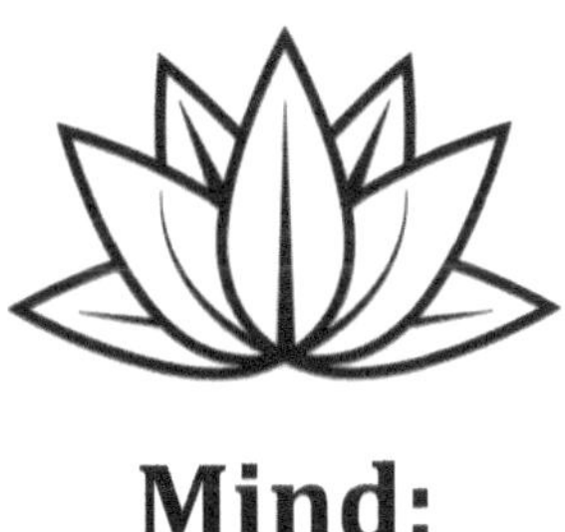

Mind:

You take it to work with you everyday

Healthy Relationships

What is a healthy relationship?

That's an interesting question. It's easy to spot when you see one, and it's even easy to recognize one when you're in it, but healthy relationships are not very easy to create intentionally. And even the best relationships are laced with their fair share of problems. If you're a part of a relationship that is not healthy, it can seem nearly impossible to improve it. And if you're hoping to get into a new relationship, there doesn't seem to be a surefire way to ensure that it stays healthy. It seems all one big game of chance. Put two people together in close quarters and just pray it goes well.

Interestingly enough, maintaining, improving and nurturing **relationships** is not something that we're ever taught. We're not taught at school. We're not really taught by our parents. And even most movies only focus on the initial stage or pursuit of a relationship. The rest is written off with a simple, "and then they lived happily ever after." But no one ever tells us exactly how that "happily ever after" is achieved. Where is the story of about the princess who has swapped out her glass slippers for therapeutic moccasins and reflects on how she and her prince managed to make it work when they couldn't pay the mortgage on the castle and the moat was flooding the basement?

Because it's never taught, chances are pretty high that your real life examples of relationships are also just blind attempts at getting it right. The only difference is that the relationships you're watching are between people who are older than you, and who you believe to have all the wisdom and answers that you don't yet have. We tend to imitate what've seen modeled to us either consciously or unconsciously. And worse, when things go south in the attempts we witness, the results affect everything we will come to believe about relationships in the future, whether true or not. Without the right resources to help us nurture and create healthy relationships, we end up with more of the same, we get stuck in old patterns that don't work, and it may never even occur to us to question the cycle.

Somehow society has perpetuated the myth that true love means two people will simply click and everything will work out. The love that the pair has for each other will conquer all. If we have chosen the correct partner or if we are sure to be "good", than our partner will naturally meet our every need. If for some reason things don't work out, it must be someone's fault.

Nothing could be farther from the truth. Relationships, much like anything else important in our lives, need constant attention and care. Most problems in a relationship are simply a matter of fault, but come from our unique ways of seeing the world. This leads to trouble communicating and understanding how to make decisions that work for both parties. This includes our workplace relationships.

It's often not uttered, but there is usually one word hovering over the relationship from the day it begins, and that word is: expectation. Both individuals enter the relationship expecting that this other person will solve every problem they ever had, they will meet every need that has gone unmet for however many years, and that they will be the one to heal every wound past, present and future.

I don't know about you but that seems like an awfully heavy load for one person to be responsible for. And interestingly, there are no other partnerships in life other than marriage where this mentality would be adopted. If you were to go into business with another person, you would both be expected to share the responsibilities. The might be different based on each person's particular strengths, but you wouldn't expect the other person to do all the work. If two people became partners in a tennis match, one wouldn't rely solely on the other to win the game. It would be a matter of teamwork. But for some reason, when we enter into a marriage, which is just another partnership, we for some reason assume that this other person will "complete" us.

But in every other endeavor we strike out on, we are already complete. Any other time we enter a partnership, whether it's with a friend or a coworker or a teammate, we enter knowing the relationship is 1 +1 = 2, but in a marriage we enter as if it is ½ + ½ = 1. As you'll see, this sets us up from the start to get hurt.

Because of this intrinsic believe that we are less than whole, we then look to the other person to complete us. We believe it is their job to soothe us in times of strife, and vice versa. This belief from the start puts us in a position of vulnerability. It says from the get-go, if we have a need, it will be unfulfilled until this other person fills it. But that other person can forget, can get busy, can withhold it, or might simply not even recognize there is a hole that needs filling. What a helpless position to put ourselves into.

We must learn that even within relationships, we must cultivate the ability to soothe ourselves. A partner is not there to fix our feelings and treat our wounds. Their presence may help. It might provide added comfort and a feeling of additional support, but that should all be in addition to the sustenance that you already have within yourself. Your worth needs to come from within. If you allow for your worth to be determined by your partner or the people around you, you're taking something you innately deserve and giving it away for other people to give back to you on their terms. It's like if you made a beautiful pitcher of lemonade on a warm sunny day, and then you gave it to another person and said, "pour me a glass of this lemonade whenever you think I deserve it." Why should that person determine when you get a glass of lemonade? You deserve to drink that juice whenever you want it. Obviously the example doesn't make much sense, and truthfully love under this strategy makes no sense either, but we still do it.

We do it because we learn that we aren't enough on our own, that we have to earn love, and oftentimes even that we should be punished for not being good enough. When others withhold love from us, we start to see the punishment as fitting. We must not have earned it. We are unlovable in some tangible way. And we should try harder to get the love we need. If only we knew, that we could love ourselves. If only we understood that the power of self-love has been tucked deep within our own hearts all along.

The big fear we struggle with as well is that if we are too deep into practicing self-care, that must mean we are neglecting our partner. A marriage means doing things together for the sake of the marriage and for the other person constantly. Only bad wives focus on meeting their own needs first. Sacrifice yourself to help others first. These are all false beliefs. There is an expression, "you can't pour from an empty cup." You literally can't. No matter how hard you try. Self-care in relationships means filling your cup first. There will be no shortage of love if you can do that. Instead it will overflow out of you, but when there is nothing to give, there is nothing to give.

Plus people tend to treat you how they see you treat yourself. Do you ever find graffiti on beautiful, well-tended houses? The answer is no. If one person cares for a place, they treat it with respect, and then others see that care, and they treat the place with respect and so on. But an abandoned building for which no cares much about, will attract endless graffiti and worse. No one seems to care about this place, so it's fine to treat it whatever way strikes your fancy at the moment. Nobody else cares, so why should an individual decide to change that. The same is true with ourselves. When you treat yourself with respect, when you take responsibility for yourself, when you take time for your mind, body and spirit, others will have no choice but to fall in line. This is not a person to mistreat. There must be something special about her because she just exudes that sense. Imagine that all that can come from just one person loving you, and that's you. When you love yourself, you set the tone for how the world should treat you.

It might also help to think about your relationships in this way. Picture the reverse. Look at your partner and imagine that their sense of worth comes only from you. You must remember to compliment them, support them, and soothe them. You must do this even if they are hiding their feelings or are scared to ask for help. You must never let your guard down, and always say the right thing or their entire self-perception will crumble. Now say, you had a tough day at work. You get home tired and exhausted, and want nothing more than to just sit down and rest for a minute so you don't notice they need an encouraging word from you.

You're just resting, but they are feeling broken, unloved and unworthy because you failed to affirm them even though it was unintentional.

Can you see from this example what an unnecessary burden you're putting on someone if everything you feel is relies on their responses or actions? Yet in relationships, we walk around with these unreasonable expectations all the time, and we are amazed when they are not met. We think that our partner is there to fix every wound we ever had in childhood. And it's these expectations that infiltrate and destroy our relationships, primarily because they are founded on unhealthy assumptions of what relationships are even for. We could stand to remember the word partnership when it comes to marriage. These feelings trickle into our workplace.

We all need to practice wellness (the practice of becoming whole), and should be able to self soothe. Only then we all be full enough of love to actually let that spill over onto the other, with no resentment, no expectation, and no strings attached.

Questions to ask Yourself

If your partner left for whatever reason, would you still feel complete?

Is your sense of worth connected to what others do or say to you?

Picture a small child. Does that child need to earn love or should the child simply be loved? Replace that child with you. Can you still see that the child deserves love no matter what?

Does your work relationships feel like a place from which you derive power and strength or is it a place where you need constant reassurance?

If you began to take some for yourself every morning and needed to not be disturbed, what kind of change would you see in your life?

Price Tag

Picture being in a bad relationship with yourself. Check off which areas of your life a bad relationship might affect.

- ❑ Work
- ❑ Children
- ❑ Other family members
- ❑ Friends
- ❑ Extracurricular activities or outside interests
- ❑ Finances
- ❑ Your sleep
- ❑ Your weight
- ❑ Your health
- ❑ Your goals/dreams
- ❑ Your faith

I think it's pretty likely that you checked off the majority of those boxes. When we are in any type of unhealthy relationship, it has a way of seeping into all the other areas of our life in one way or another.

What's the cost of all those repercussions? For simplicity's sake, let's try to measure the cost over one year. So if you were in a bad work relationship for one year, and it took its toll in the worst way on every one of these areas of your life, that would be the cost. Some of these don't have any monetary value, but we'll designate a number.

- ❑ Work – let's be modest and say $75k
- ❑ Children – they've got to be worth more than your job, so $300k
- ❑ Other family members - $150k
- ❑ Friends - $100k
- ❑ Extracurricular activities or outside interests - $10k
- ❑ Finances – finances wrecked due to marital strife are no picnic - $25k
- ❑ Your sleep – it's more important than you think and probably affects all of the above, so $30k
- ❑ Your weight – this will affect your health regardless of which direction your weight moves, so $30k
- ❑ Your health, this is huge, $50k
- ❑ Your goals/dreams, $50k
- ❑ Your faith, I'd like to say priceless, but for the sake of the math, $80k

That adds up to $900,000 for just one year.

Now does it seem like mindfulness and emotional wellness in regards to relationships need to be a priority?

That's just one area of your life and how it sends its tentacles into so many other areas especially when it's unhealthy.

What will you do now differently to keep the emotional and mental wellness whole?

Living Your Purpose

We are all here on this earth for a reason. We are not here by chance. We are not here as a mistake. We are here to bring something that only we can bring. It can be as simple as bringing a sense of humor or offering a helping hand. It can be the work that we do or the lessons that we've learned and shared, but regardless what it is, it literally can only be done by us.

As flawed people and individuals, we get busy. We get tired, and we can fall asleep to our real purpose here, but it's important for both ourselves and for the world at large that we continue to remind ourselves of our higher purpose and work on bringing that purpose forward in the world.

What I know to be true is that our purpose can absolutely not be fulfilled if we are not taking the time to care for ourselves and to meet our own needs. Avoiding self-care and taking the time to nurture our souls, our bodies and our minds is essential if we want to fulfill our purpose in the world. And the truth is, when we are working on this higher mission, we literally feel better. We have more energy because we have a destination and a goal.

Any of us can choose at any time to simply skate through life. We can settle into a state where we don't look too hard at things. We can comfort ourselves by mitigating the discomfort but not really creating any change or affecting any lives. And lots of people opt for this road. They try to placate that uneasy feeling by overeating or drinking or medicating or any number of things. Because if you can't feel, you can't recognize that you're not living your true purpose. You can just bide your time and not put up too much of a fuss.

But this doesn't do any good for you, your family or the world at large. We are an interconnected community, a social species, who lift each other up as much as we bring each other down. That is why purpose is so important. It is our contribution to the group. I think when we are not living our true purpose, we tell ourselves that our contributions don't matter much to the group. But imagine if you were going to a potluck gathering. Would you consider showing up without bringing an entrée of some sort?

I doubt it. The people at that gathering are relying on everyone to bring an item that they make best. When all the food is spread on the table, it feeds everyone in attendance, and the variety that is achieved by everyone bringing their best item is what makes the meal so beautiful. Life is the exact same way, but for some reason, we tend to get it in our heads that what we bring is not really necessary or that it doesn't really matter. For some reason, we think that when we just stay home, the party will go on fine without us. And it will go on, but it is so much improved when everyone shows up because every person invited adds something that no one else can add.

Sometimes it can be difficult to identify what your purpose even is. It might not be obvious or you might have been stuffing your strengths down for so long, that you can't even remember what's special about your contributions, but trust me, your purpose is present. It's present from the day you were born, but somewhere along the way, it has gotten lost.

When we take the time to really practice wellness and nurture our mind, body and spirit with diligence, we can reconnect with that essence, that tiny part of us that sees the world in a totally unique way. No matter who you are, there are things that only you can bring to the table, and the world is a worse place when you keep those things hidden.

You've really got to know yourself and value yourself before you can truly live your purpose. Some of us know from as early as we can remember what we are meant to bring forth in the world, but the majority of us go through lots of struggles before we really see the truth and can zero in our purpose here. It's about trusting your abilities and giving yourself the space to learn and to become open to possibility.

Maybe your purpose is in your job, or maybe you learn that your job is actually getting in the way of your purpose. This can be a real awakening and quite scary. After all, you might have spent your life working toward where you are in your career only to find that it's in conflict with who you really are. In cases like that, you have to be smart and mindful, and change your trajectory with intention and grace. But the first step is recognizing your purpose. If your job is not inline with that, it's important to realign. A soul-sucking job is no help to anyone.

Your purpose might be something you do outside of your job. It might be a hobby or cause that you believe in. Or maybe it's something less social and more personal. Maybe it's working as a mentor or helping people one on one in some way. Maybe it's your words written in the pages of a book or arranged into a song or poem. Maybe you're great at making a stranger's day brighter or maybe your only mission is to raise your children. It really doesn't matter what you discover your purpose is, only that you follow through with it.

But if you feel like you're on the wrong path or that things are going in a direction where you're not able to be your best self, you've got to move. You've got to change. Staying in toxic situations destroys your purpose and fights against it at very turn, leaving you feeling chronically defeated and unfulfilled.

The world needs all of us living our best life. There is plenty of pain and suffering. We don't need more of that. We need people living their purpose and improving the world one person at a time.

"The world is full of nice people. If you can't find one, be one." Rumi

Questions to ask yourself

Is your day filled with empty obligations that only tire you out?

What are the things in your daily life that make you feel good from within?

Is your life set up in a way that you can do more of these things on a daily basis or do you more often feel stifled?

Does it feel like you're here for some reason? And if so, how is that coming along?

What is the most important thing to you?

Do the daily tasks of your life keep that thing as a focal point?

Price Tag

If you're not living your **purpose**, what does it cost? First off, what does it cost you? I think it's safe to say, that if you're not living your purpose, it's going to affect the same areas of life that not caring for your relationships will affect. So let's say $900K again. But there's more because if you're not living your purpose, that also means that no one else in the world is reaping the benefits of what you have to offer. That special something that you bring to the world is hidden. So in essence, this price tag is multiplied.

Let's just say that you your purpose is sharing your story with others who have similar stories and inspiring them. Maybe if you talked about it at a conference of 100 people, it would help those 100 people take a step in improving their lives. So let's say that seed of growth is worth a modest $100 to each person. That's then already worth $10,000.

What if you could share that same story in a webinar and affect 10,000 people like you. Then the cost is $1 million.

The price you pay of neglecting your person is very easily near

$2 million. That's got to be an incentive to take a look in the mirror change your trajectory if you're on the wrong path.

Employee, I know your self-worth is priceless, but 2 million could easily quantify the price paid for neglecting purpose.

Thoughts?

Employers, how are you assisting in mending this gap?

Stress Reduction

Stress is now one of the leading causes of health problems in the United States, and it's not difficult to understand why. Everything about the way our society is set up contributes to increased stress. We have busy and demanding jobs that ask us to work long hours and encourage us to climb ladders by exerting ourselves to the max. Generally, the harder you work, the more you are respected. Our culture is all about success, climbing ladders and breaking barriers. Just think about who our culture naturally respects more: the CEO who puts her children in daycare so she can dedicate long hours to the office and break fiscal goals year after year or the woman who teaches yoga so that her schedule is flexible enough that she can be present for her children while still earning a decent income and having time for a balanced life?

On top of the demanding jobs, our children have demanding schedules. Remember they are being coached to join this dog-eat-dog world where winning and money are the measures of success. Our kids have more after school activities and appointments than we ever did as kids. Even their playtime is scheduled in the form of playdates. As parents, we are managing these schedules for them and are often the chauffeurs to all of these events. Oftentimes aging parents add another caveat to our schedules and responsibilities. With things like medical bills and student loans, many of us have financial burdens to shoulder and feel as though we don't have the luxury of time to waste. Some of us might try to defray those financial burdens by going back to school, and that too is fraught with more stress, demanding schedules, and more loans.

In addition to these physical causes of **stress**, there are also many emotional causes that are often swept away or pushed out of our minds, but they continue to do their work on us. Emotional stress can take its toll if we don't deal with it. Things like tough relationships, abuse, current or in the past, deaths and chronic anxiety all reek havoc on our system. It can seem like everything is a trade-off and there is little we can do to eliminate the resulting stress.

But stress must be prioritized. It is a vicious and pernicious killer. The dangerous part about stress is our body's ability to adapt to it. We trick ourselves into thinking that we're managing our stress when we are really just stuffing it down or moving it out of our consciousness. But moving stress doesn't eliminate it. It is still there doing it's damage.

So what damage is it doing exactly? After all, isn't stress a natural coping mechanism that helps us deal with high pressure situations?

This is true. Our body is uniquely prepared to deal with high stress situations. In times of stress, the brain automatically releases chemicals that trigger our fight or flight response. Adrenaline and cortisol are released by the adrenal glands. These chemicals cause our heart rate to accelerate, our blood pressure to rise, for glucose to become more accessible and for our immune response to be subdued. You can see how these are great and helpful things if we are confronted by a bear on our walk through the woods. We've now got the resources we need on hand to run, fight, stay alert and survive. But when these chemicals are getting released daily because our jobs are high pressure, our schedule is overloaded and a mountain of responsibility is resting on our shoulders, it's east to see how these same life-saving responses can go from saving us to killing us.

The scope of damage that stress does to our bodies is large and encompassing. Chronic stress has been proven to lead to cancers, heart attacks, ulcers, strokes, asthma, widespread inflammation and even fibromyalgia. Stress is tough on our digestive system, arguably the most important organ system in determining our overall health. It affects what nutrients the intestines absorb and how quickly food moves through the intestinal tract. Stress also increases the likelihood of psychological problems. Depression, anxiety, phobias and panic attacks all go up when chronic stress is in the picture.

To give you an analogy, stress is like a rocky pothole-ridden road. Our bodies are like the tires on our cars. Tires, like our bodies are pretty resilient. It's amazing how much damage a human body can actually bear. But the more stressful the life, or the more debris-ridden the road, the less resilient the body and the tires become. You can drive a long way on those tires, but eventually the stress gets to be too much, the tires become too weak, and before you know it, you've got a serious problem.

Unfortunately, there is very little we can do about how much stress is present in our lives just like we cannot take responsibility for the state of the roads. It might be nice and beneficial for our health to retreat to an island and write off all of our responsibilities, but for most of us, life simply doesn't work that way. However, there are things that we can control and measures that we can take to make sure that our stress doesn't start running our lives and breaking down our bodies. Especially at work. Do you take your breaks?

First, let's commit to daily stress reduction. One vacation a year is not enough to undo the constant, subtle affects of stress accumulated over time. Every day, we need to commit to small stress-relieving practices. We need to take control of our schedules and stop overcommitting ourselves. If we can learn to set healthy boundaries for ourselves and for our children, we will eliminate the unnecessary stress that comes as a byproduct of overcommitting. There is only so much time in a day, and we've got the same amount of hours as everyone else. We need to be reasonable for what we to commit to in a day. In our current society, it can feel like productivity at any cost is revered and laziness is demonized, and that we must do more and more if we are to be respected. But the true gold is in not necessarily doing more, but in finding more meaning in less.

For example filling your calendar with endless appointments and commitments to help out at school, pick up an extra work assignment, take an extra course, cook an extra dinner for an ailing friend and stop at one more store for supplies is not necessarily the best use of your time. If you could find a way to do just one or two of the things that are really important and then do them really well, you will not only find that the tasks are more fulfilling, but you will feel better in your body. It is better to operate at 100% for two tasks than it is to operate at 50% for seven tasks.

Next we need to set aside time for a **mindfulness practice**, whether it is mediation or a designated time for prayer. We require quiet time with just ourselves. We'll talk about this in more detail later, but even as little as five minutes per day can have enormous benefits. If your mind is constantly racing or you feel as though you are in a constant state of hyper-vigilance, you are keeping yourself in a state of arousal that is unhealthy. **Meditation** can help teach you to clear your mind, let things be, and re-focus on what's truly important.

Physical exercise is also important in managing stress. A thirty-minute walk around the neighborhood can do amazing things when it comes to the body and stress. Because stress affects the muscles and unconsciously causes tension, pain and soreness, your body might physically hurt when you are stressed. Simply partaking in some light exercise can defray this pain. It will help you relax, loosen your muscles and improve blood flow.

It's also important to commit to building a supportive network of friends and family around you. Stress is exacerbated when you are the only one bearing the weight of your struggles. Talking life through with trusted confidantes and sharing your burdens rather than suffering alone can reduce stress and offer other, often refreshing perspectives on the problems and anxieties circling in your mind. When you can share what's causing you stress with others, you may find that they can offer you ideas you hadn't thought about, support that makes you feel less alone and joy that puts things into perspective.

Questions to Ask

Do you have a strong support network around you or do you feel like you're the only one holding everything together?

Do you regularly take time for yourself each day? It doesn't have to be a lot, but can you find 5-10 minutes that is strictly for you?

Can you recognizer the symptoms of chronic stress in your body? How is it showing up for you?

What are the parts of your life and schedule that you simply cannot change? What are the commitments that you can release from your life and let go of?

Priceless Tag:

Journal here as to what stress reduction would do/change in your life?

25

Employers: How do you plan to optimize your workforce via purpose?

Time Management

As you may have noticed, a big piece of stress reduction is related to **time management.** When we don't have a good way to manage our time, we can easily become overburdened, exasperated and stressed. And as we just went through, this can lead to a whole host of health and psychological problems. How then can we manage our time in a way where we don't feel like we are managing yet another thing?

The trick is to come up with something that works for you. I'll be honest, not every time management tip and trick works for everyone. Some of us buy countless planners and find them empty and abandoned at the end of the year. Some commit with much excitement to a new app that will help keep you organized, and slowly forget about it as the days wear on. We buy giant dry erase calendars for our homes, set custom alerts on our phones, and write to-do lists on errant papers all around our offices and homes. Some things stick; most don't, and we are left feeling as inundated and strained as ever. Ultimately, we waste a lot of energy trying out the latest recommendations because we imagine it will transform our lives.

The trick of time management is much like dieting or starting a new exercise regimen. On both topics, there are thousands of books and techniques to try. They tell you everything you tried before was wrong, and you should be doing it some new way. And because you need it so badly, whether it's the secret to productivity or to weight loss, you jump in with both feet and try it. But more often than not, the book gets abandoned, the technique gets forgotten and you are no more productive or fit than you were when you started.

My belief is that the problem isn't in any particular technique but in the scope of the solution. These "solution-oriented" books and plans tend to focus on big, life-altering changes that you not only need to make, but need to maintain. And that's where the problem lies. Anything in your life that you do, and then learn to do well, you start small. You slowly integrate the thing into your life and make it a habit through small, nearly imperceptible changes rather than dramatic leaps. If you decide you want to take up the piano, you don't show up at the piano teacher's house and learn to play a composition by Mozart. You sit down and learn the keys and then you learn one chord. You practice this chord relentlessly until you know it by heart. Once you've got this down, you move onto the next chord.

The same slow integration is true for time management. Do one thing to start. Make that thing a habit. Maybe, for example you are very bad at answering emails. You read them right away and then get busy and forget to respond. Because of this you end up leaving important emails unanswered, missing opportunities for new clients and upsetting existing clients. The inclination might be to toss everything you're currently doing out the window and adopt a whole new plan in order to create a whole, new, organized you. After all if you take dramatic action, you'll likely see dramatic results. You might, but I can assure you, that you won't create lasting change.

Instead change the most important things to solve this first problem. Why not set aside a certain time of day to designate to answering emails. If you read any when they come in and they seem important, flag that email so that even though it shows up as "read," you know that you still need to take some action with it. Then do this for a week or two or three, until it becomes a part of your schedule. Then when you've got your email process squared away, move onto something else. Maybe it's finding a method of organizing everything. Some people prefer physical planners and notebooks; others like to keep everything digital in Google Calendars or some other software that will alert them to appointments and meetings. Commit to small things, make them part of your routine and then add something else when you're ready. Do this for a year and you'll see dramatic changes when you look back. But if you attempt to do a huge makeover in one week, chances are all your good intentions will be long forgotten in a few short months.

Also start to understand what is reasonable to take on and what is overextending. We touched on this in the last chapter, but it's critical to set some healthy boundaries for yourself in this department. Managing your time well does not mean stuffing everything in and celebrating when you can find a way to make it all fit. If you're putting clothes away in your dresser drawer, it's not somehow better to fit all the shirts in one drawer no matter what. If you then try to open it and it gets stuck, and you can't even see what's in there, it's not a technique that worked for you. It's one that's creating more problems. Instead you want to spread the clothes out in an organized way throughout all the drawers, so that getting dressed in the morning is easy and efficient.

Your calendar is the same way. Cramming a ton of tasks into one day is not success. What's reasonable to get done in a day? In a week? In a month? Space things out. Schedule complementing tasks together. If you have a client to see who lives close to your dentist, schedule those for the same day. If you know your kids have a busy schedule on a particular day, mark yourself unavailable to new client consults that you know are more taxing than meeting with people you already know. Be respectful of yourself. There is time to get everything done. Allow yourself time for mistakes, traffic and unforeseen events. Be generous with yourself.

And approach your schedule and your time management with a spirit of both rigidity and flexibility. It's one thing to be true to your word and to keep your commitments, but there is no need to be so strict with your schedule that it's set in stone. Allow for flexibility as well this rigidity because things will happen. The weather will throw you a curveball. Your child will get sick. The car will get a flat tire. Approaching your schedule with a mindset that embodies both rigidity and flexibility will help you manage that. You can be conscientious and generous at the same time. Conscientious to do the things you say you will do, to let people know when things change and to consider that others are managing crazy schedules too and deserve for their time to be respected, and generous enough to know when you got it wrong, when it's okay to change something, and when there's no room for another thing on that particular day.

Time management is an art when you get it right. It can so easily slip out of your control and feel like the circumstances of your life our dictating your day. It's 100% up to you remain in control. Focus on the small things that make a big impact, and embody both rigidity and flexibility when it comes to your schedule. If you can do those two things, everything else will fall into place. And remember that at the core of time management rests self-respect. Sometimes it may feel like you are Wonder Woman as you watch all the things you can accomplish in a day, but you're not. And you're not expected to be. And if some days require a lot from you, balance that out with a day that requires a little bit less. It will all get down. I promise.

Questions to Ask

Do you feel like you never have enough time?

What are you currently doing to manage you time and how is it working?

What is the biggest struggle you have when it comes to time management and productivity? What's one small thing that can help alleviate this problem?

Are you approaching time management with a respect for yourself? (If this is hard, think about what you would expect of others – would you expect someone else to squeeze in a task for you when you know they are driving all across the state that day and are maxed out – probably not, but you might tend to self –sacrifice and allow yourself to do something you would never ask of someone else. Look at that.

Priceless tag:

Take a moment to jot down your new time management system.

What changes do you expect to see in every area of your life?

Travel

Burnout is real. Our jobs tend to consume us. We have vacation days to take, but you'd be amazed at how many of those vacation days go unused at the end of the year. I've even heard people bragging about how many unused vacation days they've accumulated.

But what's amazing about unused vacation days is how little good they are doing accumulating in a employee logbook somewhere. What that number should really be telling you is how much stress you're hiding somewhere. Those days stand for days that you didn't rest, days that you didn't recharge and days where you stretched yourself just a little bit more without a break. We as Americans tend to wear those days like a badge of honor, but they are nothing to be proud of.

No one's saying that you can't do it, that you can't get through a whole year without taking one vacation day. I know you can. I know we all can. The real question is why should we? And I don't say that from a perspective of laziness or entitlement, like we've got them and we'll get paid for them, so might as well take what's ours. I'm speaking from a purely self-care focused stance. We do our minds, bodies and spirits absolutely no good by forgoing our vacation days to prove our commitment to hard work.

You can be a hard worker who takes a vacation every year. You can be a hard worker who prioritizes your vacation each year. You can even be a hard worker who looks forward to her vacation each year. And dare I say it, if you've got the days, you can even take more than one vacation a year. I'm also willing to bet that those of us who are taking our vacations are coming back better, more efficient, more refreshed, and more in tune with their purpose than those who are slogging through day after day watching their vacation days pile up.

Travel is an important part of self-care because it allows us to create space that we normally don't have a chance to create. It's great and vital to make room for the daily practices of taking time to ourselves, but travel takes that a step further. When we travel, we allow ourselves to fully disconnect. Our environment is different, our routines our different and our mindset is different.

You might say something like, "I don't need to travel. I can simply stay home for my vacation days and I won't follow my routine." You can do this. Of course. But traveling to a destination automatically takes you out of your routine. It changes everything around you. Regardless of how good your intentions are, when you are home, you will gravitate to your routines even if you are not working. Your phone or computer will seem to beckon you, the cleaning will need doing, dinner will need making, and the porch will need sweeping. When you travel, you are automatically lifted out of everything that is familiar. There will be no old habits or ingrained routines to disturb you.

You might even find that you treat yourself better when you are on vacation. We've all experienced that boost in mood when we're on a trip in some tropical location. The sun looks a little brighter, the weather feels a little sweeter and life seems a little better. You might find it easier to treat yourself to a nice meal or splurge on something you normally wouldn't. And that's all good. That's all amazingly healthy.

It's absolutely essential for our spirits to be treated with a sense of abundance, and travel provides the perfect backdrop for this. Traveling is a fun and worthwhile way to heal and reset. When we do it right, we come back refreshed and recharged, ready for anything life can throw at us. Travel literally makes us stronger. Not to mention it helps relieve the stress we talked about in a big way, a way that can't really be totally dissolved through the smaller daily practices alone.

I know that you're probably thinking that this all sounds great. "Of course, I would travel," you're thinking, "but the bills, the rent, the loans are all more of a priority than traveling." I understand that for sure. Traveling seems great in practice, but when you've got responsibilities, you've got to put travel on the backburner. After all, if you splurge on travel when you can't even make ends meet, you're just going to stress yourself out and reek havoc on your health.

I would still push back even if you do have responsibilities and financial strain. Travel doesn't have to be expensive to be satisfying or to be healthy. There are plenty of travel options that you can do on a shoestring. We can use our networks and our support systems to find cheaper alternatives to luxury vacations. You can take your week and spend it with your girlfriend in Arizona. No one is telling you that you need to stay in a fancy hotel on an exotic island for it to count as a vacation. You only need to change the scene, go somewhere that is new for you, and you can absolutely go with friends or family who can split costs.

The payoff of making travel a priority regardless of your financial situation is the mental, physical and spiritual benefits that this time away provides you with. There is no substitute for a week away where you don't have to think about anything other than what relaxing thing you're going to do next.

And make it a digital detox as well. Leave your phone and email behind, and if you can't manage that, then at least allocate a portion of each day to be technology-free. You'll be amazed at what disconnecting from your email feels like. And I guarantee you it's possible for everyone in your world to survive without email access to you for a week. Just a couple of decades ago, this was a common occurrence, but we've become so linked to our phones in the past decade that we can't remember that time. It seems unfathomable. But trust me, everything will be okay.

Questions to Ask

When was the last time you took a vacation?

How many unused vacation days do you have? Are you collecting them or do you use them regularly?

Have you ever done a digital detox, in which you stopped checking your phone for a period of time?

Pick a place you would love to travel to this year.

Priceless tag:

Write out your thoughts here regarding the answers to the questions above.

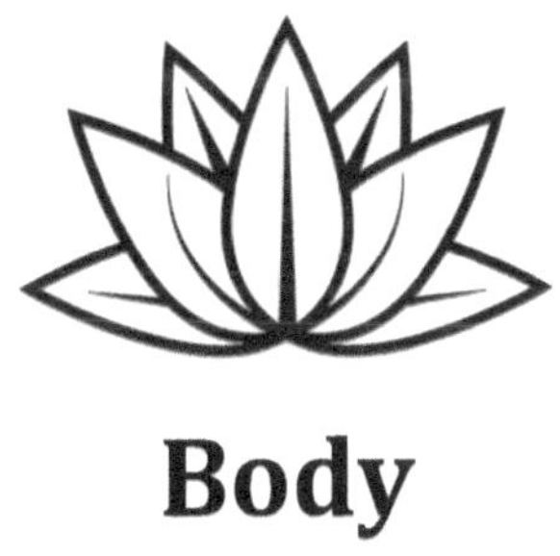

Body

It travels with us everywhere that we might go......
and will be our only home

Exercise

We have bodies because we are meant to move them. There are two ways to think of our bodies. We can look at them as a burden placed upon us. After all, it's our bodies that feel pain, our bodies get tired, they fail us, they disappoint us, they require feeding and grooming and upkeep of all sorts. When you see your body in this way, exercise feels like a chore or just another thing to fit into our schedule.

Alternatively, we can view our bodies as tools. Our body is a set of tools that our mind and spirit have to work with to get things done in the world. And under that view, we can look at our bodies and see what a gift or what a great resource to do our work. When we see our bodies in this way, then we can more easily understand that exercising and moving the bodies aren't more tasks we need to fit into our day. Instead our body is a way for us to make sense of the world.

By that definition, exercise is one of the most potent activities we can do to improve our lives. Even simple forms of exercise like walking around the neighborhood has the power to boost our mood, reduce stress, improve our sleep, increase our metabolism and help us manage our weight. But even more than that, exercise helps us switch gears. It helps us clear our mind, and in those times of clarity, we make connections we couldn't make if we were immersed in work. A brisk walk can help you think of new solutions to old problems, it will spark your creativity and charge you up with more energy than you had when you started.

Many of us feel a decline in energy around 3pm in the afternoon, and we tend to think a coffee run is the cure for the energy lull, but you could replace that afternoon coffee with a twenty minute walk and you'll feel twice as good.

I'm sure you've experienced the mental changes that I'm talking about that you can get from exercising. You're out for a walk and suddenly an idea strikes you seemingly out of nowhere or you're on the treadmill at the gym and suddenly, you have a new perspective on what your husband was saying to you the night before. These flashes of creativity or inspiration come to us during exercise because our mind never really stops working on problems, but when we are actively thinking about something, we are using our frontal lobe. When we exercise, the frontal lobe is no longer on center state. Our mind is wandering, we're focusing on our breathing and our body, so our mind has the ability to leap all over the place, thus resulting in divine flashes of inspiration.

Exercise causes our bodies to release endorphins or the "feel-good" hormones, so a half hour of exercise makes us feel good for no other reason than that we have moved our bodies. The more you make a habit of exercise, the more often you will feel good. You'll see results in your muscle tone, you'll probably slim down a bit, and sure enough, you'll start to increase your self-confidence. This is true whether you're confident already or not. Whatever your current state is, you will feel even better when you exercise regularly. Because your body feels strong, your spirit will feel strong.

I know that even as I praise the benefits of exercise, lots of you are thinking to yourself, "that's all great, but I don't have the time." It might seem that so many things have to be moved ahead of exercise in a day, that although it all seems like a really nice goal, it's hardly feasible. If the weather is too cold for walking where you are, you might cringe at the idea of signing up for a gym membership. Another monthly withdrawal from your checking account just means more stress, it's another thing to fit into your schedule, and then it's guilt if you can't get there and now you're paying for membership you don't use. Just thinking about it is stressful.

I understand all of your hesitations, and for some of us, more than others, exercise can seem very intimidating. We might have an ingrained belief that exercise is just not for us, we've never been athletic, and it's silly to start now. But exercise doesn't have to be something dramatic. I'm not asking you to join a professional team or to train like you're headed for the Olympics. Exercise can be anything that you enjoy as long as your body is moving. For some, brisk walking is ideal. Others might enjoy the idea of swimming or yoga or a group class at a gym. Maybe you feel more at home on a bicycle on a beautiful local trail or hiking in the woods. Whatever you enjoy, get out and do it.

And if you have trouble keeping yourself motivated, you can solicit a friend to go on this journey with you. This can prove to be doubly helpful as you're both getting some physical exercise and making time for connection. These two things are both great stress relievers. And of course when you have an exercise buddy, you've taken care of accountability and will both be more likely to follow through on your new habit.

Another objection I've heard from women is guilt. They feel guilty making time for their own exercise routines when they have families at home that need them. This guilt might feel like it's coming from a healthy, caring place, but putting your health and your exercise routine first is not selfish. You are worth more to your family if you are healthy, strong and energetic than if you are constantly sacrificing your own body so that you can be there for them. Exercise improves mental focus and increases productivity, so taking the time to exercise means that you will be better equipped to provide and nurture than you will be if you skip caring for your body.

If you're feeling overwhelmed or stuck trying to make up your mind about what form of exercise you should partake in, just choose. It doesn't matter what you choose, it just matters that you're doing something, especially at the start. If later you realize that you're doing plenty of cardio and want to tone your muscles a bit, you can add that in, but initially the most important thing is to start. Try not to get stuck in overthinking. Do what comes the most naturally for you. And do something that you can look forward to, not something that creates anxiety or fear.

Some people think that a group class is the way to go, but learning aerobics steps in front of a mirror with a bunch of strangers elicits only fear and anxiety in them. They have to mentally prep for hours or days before they can get the courage up to go to class. Don't choose something like this. Choose an activity that is right for you, and not something that you think will have the best results. All forms of exercise are beneficial, so you don't have to force yourself into something that doesn't fit. If nothing seems more boring to you than a walk or run around the neighborhood, don't make that your plan. You're only going to stick with it if its something you enjoy, so make sure you enjoy it.

Once you start making exercise a regular part of your daily routine, you're going to see benefits that go beyond the physical. Yes, your body will feel better, but you'll also feel your mood brighten. Your stress will decrease. You'll gain confidence. You'll be getting a better night's sleep, and you'll be feeling strong, energized and ready to conquer the world. Just take the first step.

Questions to Ask:

Do you currently make it a priority to exercise? How many times a week are you currently active?

Do you have low energy? Do hit a wall in the late afternoon?

What are your preconceptions about exercise and do you see yourself as someone who is fit or who has to potential to be fit?

Do you have habits that you resort to that leave you feeling down that you can replace with exercise?

Priceless Tag:

The costs of sedentary living makes the red arrow point up.

Employees, what changes do you expect to see after reading this chapter?

Employers, how to you expect to share the gift of exercise with your workforce?

Nutrition

We talked about exercise and how important it is. But exercise could never even be achieved if it weren't for nutrition. The food we eat is what gives us the energy to do absolutely everything. As I'm sure you know, our bodies can't go long without food, and they can go even less time without water. Every thought, every breath, every step, is only possible because of food. And it's the quality of that food that determines how well our body functions for us.

An entire book can be written solely on diet, and there are plenty out there. I'm not here to tell you which diet is right for you or what foods make the most sense for your body. Some people will tell you not to eat meat; others swear by it, still others swear only by ethically-raised meat. Some people will tell you to avoid gluten or carbs or sugar. Eat whole grains, don't eat any grains, limit your fat, eat a lot of fat. There are no shortage of messages out there, and many of them are conflicting.

I think that the most important message for you to adopt is to simply eat a variety, and to eat as little processed food as you can. If you focus on keeping a rainbow of colors on your plate, buying real ingredients as often as possible, and keeping your splurging to minimum, you'll do just fine.

Another good tip to improve nutrition without going on a crazy diet is to plan out your meals with intention. Pack your lunches the night before, make a grocery list of meals for the weak every Sunday and then shop based on that list, and even create a food journal where you record what you're eating daily. When you are mindful about planning what you eat, you will naturally tend to eat a little better. Think about it. When you take the time to plan out what lunches you will take to work the night before, you will be more thoughtful about what you choose. You can make yourself salads full of your favorite veggies, hard boiled eggs, and grilled chicken. You can include some healthy snacks to eat during the day, and you can do this all in a way that promotes using everything in your fridge so items don't go bad.

If you wait until you're at work and starving before you give any thought to what you're going to eat that day, you're going to end up going to the closest fast food restaurant to the office. And because you're so hungry, you are extra likely to overeat. The same is true for dinners. When you don't plan them out ahead of time, you tend to be already hungry when you're making your decision. Suddenly your chance of abandoning any inclination to cook a well-balanced meal and opting for takeout increases exponentially.

Mindfulness in eating is really so important. Simply writing down what you eat in a day will make you more aware of your choices. And because we, as humans tend to be judgemental and particularly hard on ourselves, we don't want to write down that we ate a sleeve of Oreos. Before you know it, you'll find that you're selecting foods more often that you feel good about writing down.

It truly does feel good to eat healthy. It even feels good to buy healthy food. It's always interesting to look at what the people around you are putting onto the checkout counter at the grocery store. And its always satisfying to see lots of fruits and vegetables, eggs, nice meats and other quality foods as you load your items onto the conveyer belt.

Plus the more healthy foods you eat on a regular basis, the less guilty you'll feel when you do actually splurge. When you're in a rut and you're eating a lot of comfort foods, you feel good in the moment, but you tend to feel really guilty right after. You're disgusted to see the empty chip bag or the plate full of cake crumbs. But when you're eating well most of the time, and you end up treating yourself to that amazing apple fritter, you don't feel bad at all. You feel like you deserved that. After all, you've been doing so well. Good nutrition changes your inner monologue to one of encouragement rather than that self-deprecating voice always warning you against the cookie and scolding you when you eat it anyway. It's time to change that story.

Eat healthy as often as you can. Treat your body with respect. Your body in turn will function better. You'll feel better. Your skin will look better. Your nails will be stronger. And even your mind will work better. Give your body what it needs, and it will reward you.

Questions to Ask:

What does your daily diet look like? How satisfying is this diet?

Do you plan your meals ahead of time or do you mostly wing it?

Are you always on a diet or always about to start a new diet?

Do you think about meals as nutrition or do you see them as something else?

What is your lifetime relationship with food like?

Price Tag

Screenings

Health screenings and annual exams are like report cards at school or progress reports at work. They are a snapshot of a period in time and an excellent way to know where you stand in terms of your health. Without understanding where you are at, it's impossible to figure out where you need to go.

Many adults neglect preventative care and annual screenings because they feel well enough. If they had a problem, they would see a doctor. That's a mentality that will work for some people some of the time. Your Uncle Earl might claim that he never went to the doctor, and rightfully so because he never had a single thing wrong with him. That's great for Uncle Earl, but chances are he was just lucky. If something had been going on with him, he would never have known in time to treat the problem.

Knowledge truly is power when it comes to your health. Big diseases and life-altering health issues don't typically appear out of thin air. You don't just get type II diabetes without there being some signs, and the symptoms that you are at risk for a heart attack are probably in the numbers long before the big heart attack hits. Of course there are always outliers and cases that defy all odds, but if you have a chance to protect against something, wouldn't you take it? Most big health issues started as small signs. And when the signs are small, that's when it's easiest to make small but powerful alterations to change course.

Elevate blood pressure can be handled long before takes its toll on the cardiovascular system. High cholesterol can be corrected before it builds up enough to cause damage. And metastasized tumors are always small tumors before they are big ones.

Beyond the benefit of testing for abnormalities, regular screening that is consistent provides a great reservoir of information for doctors and nurses to work with. When there is a collection of information from years of annual screenings, it is easier for doctors to spot patterns and identify what is out of the norm for your particular body. More information is rarely ever a problem. When doctors can look at a comprehensive sample of your past records, they are better informed and can more easily distinguish what is normal for you and what is important to analyze deeper. After all, what is alarming in one patient can be absolutely normal in another.

Many people cite fear as a reason that they stay out of doctors' offices. They'd rather not know than be presented with news that is scary or difficult to deal with. This is an understandable way to feel, but we've got to move past our fears and take ownership of our bodies. It might be scary to hear that something is wrong or that we need to make a change, but it is lot less scary to hear this news when there is still something you can do about it.

When you wait to too long to take action, you are actively taking options off the table. Yes every time you go for a mammogram, you're going to worry that something will show up on the scans. And you can easily avoid that fear by skipping those mammograms. This avoidance might end up being the difference between having a lumpectomy and changing your diet to having a full mastectomy, chemo and radiation. That's a big difference.

The thing to hold onto when it comes to facing your fears and being diligent about screenings is that you are putting yourself in position to be your own advocate when you take control of your health. Be diligent. Insist on more information. And encourage the loved ones around you to take ownership of their health as well. When you have a full picture of your health, you can make smarter decisions for you body. If you know you are prone to high blood pressure or high cholesterol or that your Vitamin D is lower than it should be, you can take actions that make sense for you. If you don't have this awareness, you don't have a road map. You don't have a clear sense of what eating healthy looks like for you in particular. You don't know what kind of exercise makes the most sense for you.

The bottom line is to be proactive when it comes to your health. In the arena of your body and your health, what you don't know can literally hurt you.

Questions to Ask

When was the last time you had a screening or preventative exam?

If you haven't been recently, what is preventing you from going?

Is it important that you are healthy for your family? Are you doing all that you can to make that a reality?

How would it burden the family if you heard bad news? Would the burden be less if you waited as opposed to finding a smaller problem was present now?

Price Tag

Sleep

Somehow this biological need has come to be a luxury that many of us think we can't afford. As a culture, we've become sleep-sacrificers, believing that trading in precious hours of sleep for more time to spend on our to-do lists, tending to others, studying extra, or squeezing some additional exercise time is the noble and honorable thing to do. We tell ourselves that our lives our simply so jam-packed with important tasks that the only option is to go to bed later or to wake up earlier. We trick ourselves into believing that we operate just fine on five hours per night and we comfort ourselves with the believe that we are supercharging our productivity and getting superhuman levels of work done in a day.

But copious studies prove that sleep is just as important if not more important than nutrition and exercise. Our bodies quite simply need sleep to function properly, and when we shortchange ourselves in this department, we are not giving our bodies the opportunity to recharge and recover in very significant ways. When we don't get enough sleep, we are likely depriving ourselves of our deep, restorative sleep. The average adult requires 7-9 hours of sleep per night, and there's no satisfactory way around this. You can't deprive yourself for days and hope that a weekend sleeping binge will catch you back up. Each day that you are sleep-deprived, your body is suffering consequences that are gradually adding up and doing damage to your health.

Even when you think you are sleep-depriving yourself for good causes, like when you wake up early to go for a morning run, you are in fact hurting your body. If you are operating on less than seven hours of sleep per night, I'd caution you against the morning run as your sleep practices are counteracting the good that you think you're doing. Sleep deprivation messes with your metabolism. Your body uses the time when you are asleep to burn fat, but this cycle gets altered when you are not consistently getting enough sleep.

Sleep deprivation also causes hormone imbalances, leaky gut and brain fog. Sleep is the body's time to reset. First, it addresses physical restoration and repairs muscles. Once that is complete, it moves on to restore the mind. This is when the days memories are sorted and moved from short-term memory to long-term memory. Your brain also works to reorganize thoughts and continues working on the problems of the day. When you deprive yourself of sleep, you prevent these processes from taking place. And when you continue to do this over the long-term, the consequences can be significant.

Long-term sleep deprivation can lead to serious health concerns like diabetes, obesity, heart disease and stroke. Most people don't give sleep this much credit. We look at it as a luxury, and we say things like, "I'll sleep when I'm dead." We somehow came to understand that sleep is a waste of time, and that sleeping in the midst of an exciting and active life is a way to escape or is simply a way of missing out on all that life has to offer. Trust me, sleeping for seven to nine hours per night will still leave you with plenty of life to experience.

Sometimes, however, sleep deprivation is not so much of a choice, but a result of other problems like anxiety, insomnia, or just poor routines. Some of us legitimately make an effort to get a healthy amount of sleep, but we simply end up tossing and turning all night long. Maybe we wake up easily or aren't sleeping soundly. Whatever the case, we must do our best to find the source of our troubles and address them. It's not enough to simply shrug our shoulders and resign to the fact that we aren't good sleepers. The consequences are too numerous and long-reaching.

There are some simple steps that we can take before we resort to seeking professional help. As we would teach and encourage our children to do, we need to also teach ourselves to adopt a period of unwinding. As bedtime approaches, start to slow down and go inward. Try not to partake in vigorous exercise during the few hours leading up to bedtime. Instead do things to slow the heart rate down like taking a bath, reading a book or listening to relaxing music. Developing a peaceful before bed routine is a great way to signal to your body that it is time for sleep, and you'll find that when this pattern becomes a habit, your body will fall asleep more easily.

It's also important to try to regulate your body's internal clock. Try to go to sleep and wake up at the same time every day, even on weekends. Oftentimes, we stay up extra late on weekends and might also sleep in the following morning. This creates a problem when Monday morning comes around again. If you slept in on Sunday morning, you'll find it much harder to fall asleep early that night so that you can wake for work on Monday. However, if you keep your sleeping as consistent as possible, you can minimize this problem.

Finding a regular and healthy sleep schedule can be especially difficult for those of us who have jobs that require us to be awake overnight. When this is the case, it's important to be extra diligent. Because natural light has such an effect on energy levels and sleep patterns, we must do all that we can to ensure that we are still getting a healthy amount of deep, nourishing sleep. In these cases, try to arrange your room so that it can be dark during the day or sleep with a mask. Also make sure that your sleep is a priority. Try not to be tempted to sacrifice this sleep for time with family and friends who are awake while you should be sleeping.

Also be familiar with how your body deals with caffeine. If you drink caffeine late in the day, it might affect your ability to fall asleep. Be observant of how your body reacts to caffeine and whether this creates problems for you. Some people can have a coffee right before bed and fall right to sleep. Others will be tossing and turning for hours. Notice how your body reacts and then adapt your habits, option for decaffeinated options and herbal teas if you like a warm beverage before bed.

Rich or high-sugar foods can also be problematic for some people. Again be cognizant about how the foods you eat affect your sleep and take actions to avoid eating these things before bedtime.

The bottom line is that quality sleep is essential to our health. It's not okay to sacrifice sleep. We think that we are being selfless or extra-productive when we skip sleep to do other things, but the truth is that we are sabotaging our good efforts. If you are healthy in every aspect of your life, and you consistently sacrifice sleep, you are sabotaging those good efforts. Your body needs sleep to burn calories, store memories, heal muscles and do other important work. Don't trick yourself into believing that your body doesn't need this time.

Questions to Ask:

How much sleep do you get on a typical night?

Do you find yourself inclined to skip sleep when you don't feel as if you have time to do a particular thing?

Do you sleep soundly through the night or do you consistently wake up throughout?

Have you struggled to make changes in your diet or exercise, but haven't seen any results? Could this be related to not getting enough sleep?

Price Tag

Water

I know this isn't the first time you've heard how important it is to drink water. Our bodies are constantly using water to carry out daily functions. Water helps us to do so many things including, flushing waste, regulating our temperature and helping our brains to function. In addition to that it also helps moisturize and hydrate everything from our skin to our joints. Without water, our bodies simply wouldn't be able to operate, which is why we can last about 30 days without food, but can't go much more than three days without water.

Yet despite knowing about all that water does and having heard this message throughout our entire lives, many of us still do not get enough water. It's very easy to opt for other, often dehydrating beverages, instead of water. We love our coffees, teas, sodas and alcoholic beverages. We find it much more satisfying or easier to drink two to three coffees a day or to sit at a bar with a friend and drink an entire bottle of wine than we do to drink our daily allotted amount of water.

There are disagreements about exactly how much water is required, and of course it varies based on the person. A petite woman would require less water than a tall, hulking football player, but still we find it very difficult to drink as much as we need. And whenever we do drink those dehydrating beverages, we really should compensate with an additional glass of water. If you have two coffees, you should add two more waters to your drinking list for the day.

But many of us claim to just not like the taste or lack of taste that water has. It's much more appealing to gulp down a glass of sweet and tangy lemonade or to splurge on an ice cold Root Beer than to opt for the plain and boring water. But even still, it remains important that we do choose water, at least most of the time. Our bodies require it, and it's a simple way to cut needless calories. A soda that is full of sugar is a fairly unsatisfying way to take in 140 calories, especially considering that you're sure to still be hungry afterwards. And even opting for a diet soda will save you the calories, but will replace them with a plethora of chemicals that your body does not need to function.

I encourage you to replace as many of your daily beverages with water as possible. Water is a healthy, calorie-free way to improve your health. If you can't stomach the plain taste, there are plenty of healthy ways to spice up your water without losing the benefits. You can try adding fruit. Citrus fruits make a simple and easy addition to any glass. You can also try adding things like mint, rosemary or basil to your water for an alternative flavor. You can also even try adding a few drops of essential oils to your water. Some popular flavors to add include, mint, orange, lemon, lime, or lavender. You could also try muddling different fruits, like blueberries, watermelon or strawberries and freezing them into ice cubes. Then use those cubes in your water for a subtle flavor infusion.

As you know alcoholic beverages are very dehydrating, but it's okay to drink in moderation. A simple way to defray the negative effects of these beverages is to alternative every boozy beverage with a glass of water. So if you drink one margarita, drink a full glass of water before you order a second margarita. Not only will this counteract the dehydrating effects of the alcohol (and help with any hangovers), it will also prevent you from overdrinking, and will cut down on the tab as well. It's a win-win.

Whatever route you take, the most important thing is to simply drink water as often as you can. You can check your urine to see whether you are dehydrated or not. If it's clear, you're on the right track, but if it's dark yellow, you are likely dehydrated. Invest in a water bottle that you can fill in the morning and drink from throughout the day. You don't have to obsess about your ounces, but the more healthy choices you make and the more you make an effort to swap out your other beverages for water, the healthier you'll be.

Questions to Ask:

How much water do you drink in a day?

What color is your urine usually?

Do you often feel thirsty?

Do you only choose water when you are exercising?

Are there instances where you could swap your current beverage for water?

Price Tag

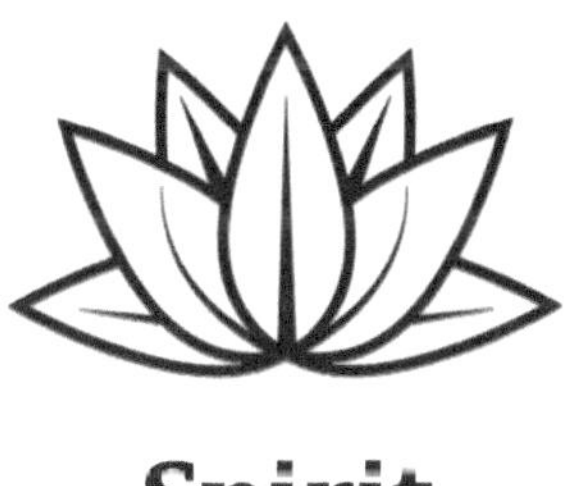

Spirit

"When you recover or discover something that nourishes your soul and brings joy, care enough about yourself to make room for it in your life." **~ Jean Shinoda Bolen**

Faith & Prayer

We've been talking about some really tangible forms of self-care for awhile now, and I want to stress the importance of all the things that have gone before. However, I also want to offer the idea of faith and prayer as your starting point. If you've been reading patiently up until now, and you haven't been completely compelled as to the importance of self-care up to this point, it might be because faith is the place to start.

If you're having trouble resonating with the idea of self-care as something that you should be doing, it might help to reframe it as something that is not yours to do. Self-care becomes easy when we understand that it is God's will. He created us in his image, and it might be easier to see ourselves as something special to Him rather than a body that we must care for in order to thrive.

From this perspective, self care is not work that we do in ourselves and for ourselves. Instead, we must create space within ourselves for God to carry out this work. If we have faith and have nurtured this faith through prayer, we understand that we are here on this earth to serve God. When we search ourselves, we understand that we have a Divine Purpose bestowed upon us by God Himself. If this faith is strong enough and unwavering, we can then begin to clearly see that self-care is not selfish. It is simply God's will wrapped up in a human body, our human body.

As humans, we are called to nurture and cultivate our faith. We must learn to trust in God's plan, and in that plan, we as individuals are important. Everything that exists in this world to heal and nurture the human body is also part of God's plan. He created us with bodies that can move and exercise. He created a world where nutrients and minerals abound in the foods that we can eat. He created water to nourish us and to help our bodies' function. You can even say he created the people who invented the screenings and who have gathered the knowledge that we can use to gauge our health and to take steps to heal ourselves.

God also created our minds and our companions on this earth. He created these things to help us, to make us stronger by working and relating to others. He placed us all here complete with strengths and weaknesses so that we could all help and learn from each other. He made the world a big place so that we could travel, explore and learn. He even gave us our current stress reaction system so that we could survive in a world that is as dangerous as it is wondrous. And he gave us some logical mental functioning so that we could prioritize and plan our lives so as to have the ability to figure out how to enjoy all of what he laid out for us.

But what He didn't do, was give us our bodies so that we can take advantage of them, treat them with disrespect, neglect them and use them thoughtlessly. He gave us this resource and he gave us a million ways to care for this resource. It is our faith that we need to employ in order to care for this gift in a loving and generous way. And when our faith falters or when the noise gets to loud, it's prayer that we can use to maintain this connection with the Divine.

So if can cultivate a strong faith and trust in God, we will automatically opt to care for ourselves and to see our bodies and minds as temples. But how can we do this? How do we cultivate a strong faith? How do we use prayer as a tool?

As human's, it's very easy to get caught up or stuck in our bodies. Our bodies are great tools, but they come with a lot of features or distractions that make it difficult to focus on our faith. You might think of it like being given a car. To make it from one destination to another, we really need only a very basic car, a Model T, will do. It needs a wheel, an engine, brakes and a gas pedal. But the cars of today are loaded with all sorts of other distractions, interactive screens, heated seats, cruise control, radios, climate control, sunroofs and any other number of features. All of these distractions make it difficult to remember that we are just moving along a path, going from here to there. We start fiddling with and obsessing over the features, and we forget where we are going, we get into accidents, we run through stop signs, and we get citations.

These distractions could be likened to the elements of personality that are our defense mechanisms or anxieties. If we were abandoned as a child, we might be sensitive to sharing attention with others or if we were pushed to be perfect, we might have a strong inner critic constantly berating us. We all have these ways of dealing with the world, and it's these distractions that make us forget that we are on a path back to God, that we were placed on this path for a reason that is bigger than ourselves and our insecurities, and that we must continue to steer the course.

That is when we need to call upon our faith. And we might need to use prayer to do so. In our prayers, we can ask for guidance when we lose our way. When we get distracted, we must find ways to refocus on our true mission and our true path. Our bodies are great inventions. God created them to be able to do everything that we need to fulfill our mission. They are created in such a way that everything around us can be used to nurture and nourish our bodies so that we can get them back in alignment to move forward with our path. But they are also very vulnerable tools at the same time. However, it is our job, given to us by God, to make sure that we continue to care for these bodies so that we can continue to do God's work here on Earth.

Our faith is why we must prioritize self-care.

Questions to Ask

How has your faith helped you on your path back to God?

When do you pray? How does it help strengthen your faith?

Have there been times when your faith has wavered?

When you are strong in your faith, do you also have a strong motivation for self-care?

Price tag

Meditation

When we picture meditation, we often picture limber spiritual gurus sitting on a special pillow with a clean and empty mind for hours at a time. With that high standard in place, we think to ourselves that mediation is surely out of reach for us. Our minds are constantly racing, and if they weren't racing, the world would surely fall apart. Whether we feel that it is our duty to be constantly thinking and planning and wondering or whether it's because we simply can't stop ourselves, meditation is an accessible solution.

Interestingly enough, the literal definition of meditation is to engage in mental exercise, which sounds an awful lot like thinking. In practice, it is closer to clearing your mind and therefore becoming more present. There are many forms of meditation that are all different to varying degrees, but one simple way to get started is to simply set aside a specific amount of time when you won't be disturbed. It can be as little as five minutes. Get seated in a comfortable position and close your eyes. Then focus on nothing other than your breathing. If your mind starts to wander, gently nudge it back to thinking only of your breath.

It might seem like on the surface, doing something this simple would be nothing but a waste of time. After all we have so much to do in a day. But in reality, this is a beneficial daily practice with positive repercussions for your body, mind and spirit. It teaches us how to sit with ourselves in the present moment. We are so often thinking about the future and the past, that we can lose sight of the present moment. And the present moment is where we gain the ability to deal with all of lives struggles.

Because the future hasn't happened yet, speculating about it, planning for it and thinking about it can only cause us worry. We don't know what is there. It is out of our reach. It's not even a surety that we will make it there. Similarly the past has already happened. It can't be changed and no amount of regret or longing can alter the things that have already happened. All we truly have is the present moment. If we can learn to be right here in this moment, then we can learn to handle anything that comes our way. Every problem, every struggle must be moved through one breath at a time.

Meditation on regular basis yields a host of benefits. It has been shown to improve attention span, body image, memory, blood pressure, and sleep. It can help to decrease pain and can help with addiction. It may even help you in extending more kindness to others. Based on what specific benefits you are looking for, you can find a mediation style that makes the most sense for you.

One of the great things about the practice is that it extremely accessible. You don't need fancy equipment or expensive courses to teach you how to do it. In fact, these days there are plenty of apps that can guide you through various meditations. You can practice meditation in your own home or anywhere else that is comfortable for you. You can even practice forms of walking or moving mediation.

Simply taking even just five minutes to yourself can have positive effects on the rest of your day. You will be able think more clearly, you will be more present in all the activities you partake in and you will have more energy to dedicate to these endeavors. Make room for mediation in your day, and you will see that your day becomes much more manageable.

Questions to Ask

Is your mind constantly racing? Do you have trouble clearing your head?

Do you often find yourself dwelling on the past or speculating into the future? Does this disrupt your daily life?

Do you ever take some quiet time for yourself to start the day or do you just jump right into the day?

Priceless Tag:

Take a moment to journal daily.

Belief in God

"You cannot believe in God until you believe in yourself"
~ Swami Vivekananda

It can be easy to think that our belief in God comes first, and then after we know God, we can then work on loving ourselves and others. But that is quite a big ask. First off, how are we to know how to love an invisible, Almighty being whom we've never seen and who we understand and believe to have created all things and is ever powerful? To scale it down a bit for understanding's sake, that's like telling the young children in your family that they need to love and respect their great-great-grandmother who's only presence is perhaps portrait at the top of the stairs. The reasoning for this might be something along the lines of, "she was an amazing woman with great morals and she is the matriarch of this family. She sacrificed her own dreams so that her children and her children's children would have a better life, and it is her values that we pass down from generation to generation so you need to embody these as well.

As great as that sounds and as important and true as that might be, it doesn't give the child much tangible information to go on as far as "how" to do that. A more productive approach might be to teach the child about themselves. You can say things like: you are kind like your great-great-grandmother; you are generous like her; you are smart like her. Then you might teach the child to recognize these same qualities in their siblings and parents and then their cousins and extended family. They would be able to practice loving themselves and their family members in ways that made sense to them. So then when they are older and you mention that matriarch and her values, they can easily relate to both her and the core family values that she passed down.

This is why is important that for us to truly love and believe in God, we must first love and believe in ourselves. The loving acts of self-care that we make a part of a daily routine are ways of loving God since we are his creations. When we neglect ourselves, we are disrespecting the gift he gave us and are moving farther away from Him.

When we look at ourselves and believe in our goodness and our power and our wisdom, we come closer to believing in God. If we look at ourselves, and we don't see anything good, we are closing our eyes to God. God didn't create junk. Unfortunately, because of some of the harsh messaging we receive, we teach ourselves to believe this falsehood. We think we are flawed or undeserving or that God somehow made a mistake. But God doesn't make mistakes. We are here and we made in his image. It is our daily mission to ensure that we don't ever forget that.

Taking the time to love ourselves, to treat ourselves with kindness and to be generous with ourselves is the path to God. We learn to love God by loving ourselves. When we love ourselves, we are better able to love others and to see that they too are creations of God. Loving others teaches us to love differences because once we learn to love ourselves, our ego might tell us that we are the only version of a person that God created. We might think if people are not like us, they must not be a creation of God or maybe they are a mistake. Again neither of those things are true.

But God doesn't' make loving others easy. Those differences that we learn to recognize create a lot of conflict. But when we work on loving those who have different opinions and different beliefs, we grow in unexpected ways. We start to see that all those differences are embodied in God and we can learn how to open our hearts to all of it.

Regardless of what specific purpose we have in this lifetime, this is a path that we all share. This is the core reason why self-care is so vital, and why it is so far from a selfish path.

Questions to Ask

How does your belief in God affect how you act in daily life?

Do you currently consider loving yourself to be equivalent to loving God?

Do you make an effort to love others even when you don't get along?

Priceless Tag:

Spiritual wellness is a part of wholeness.

How does your workplace make room for spiritual health/ observances?

Conclusion

In conclusion, I hope that you able to see how deeply important wholeness and wellness truly is. We need to be diligent with caring for ourselves, not only to help others and to respect ourselves, but to truly appreciate the power of God's gift to us. The rage that we feel when we see injustice in the world or bullies taunting and hurting the weak, should be just as present when we notice ourselves neglecting our bodies or stressing our minds. What is easy to witness in the world at large is tough to see in ourselves, but we must do our part. We must look within ourselves for our true essence and then we must nurture that being. That is truly the only way that good can happen in the world and in the workplace.

This book is truly only a starting point for self-care. There are many resources available to you if you struggle in one or more particular areas. Often we don't neglect every area. Some of us are great at exercise, but we don't sleep. Others meditate and pray, but continue to stay in unhealthy relationships. Still others seem to check off all the boxes, but never say no to an engagement or take a vacation.

Learn to understand that the entire picture of self-care is necessary in order to live your best life. If you are struggling in one area, you are likely suffering. And according to God's will, you needn't be. We are all here struggling with similar demons, but it is through true self-care that we can push past these demons and find grace with God and peace within ourselves.

And it's okay to forget these things from time to time. The trick comes in learning to notice when you are slipping off the path and not paying enough attention. That's when it's helpful to pick this book back up and revisit it. Notice what healthy routines you fell out of and what unhealthy tendencies you picked up. There is always room to switch gears and to get back on the path to God.

I hope that this book has opened some doors and helped shed some light on what is happening in your life and where you can start to make a change.

To engage in deeper work, I offer one-on-on coaching to support you on your path.

I look forward to hearing from you on your wellness journey and how it has changed/affected your career/workplace.

Email me at : support@greenerhodesconsulting.com

Or visit me for Consultation

at www.greenerhodesconsulting.com